Workbook

Home Health Aide Textbook

Home Care Principles

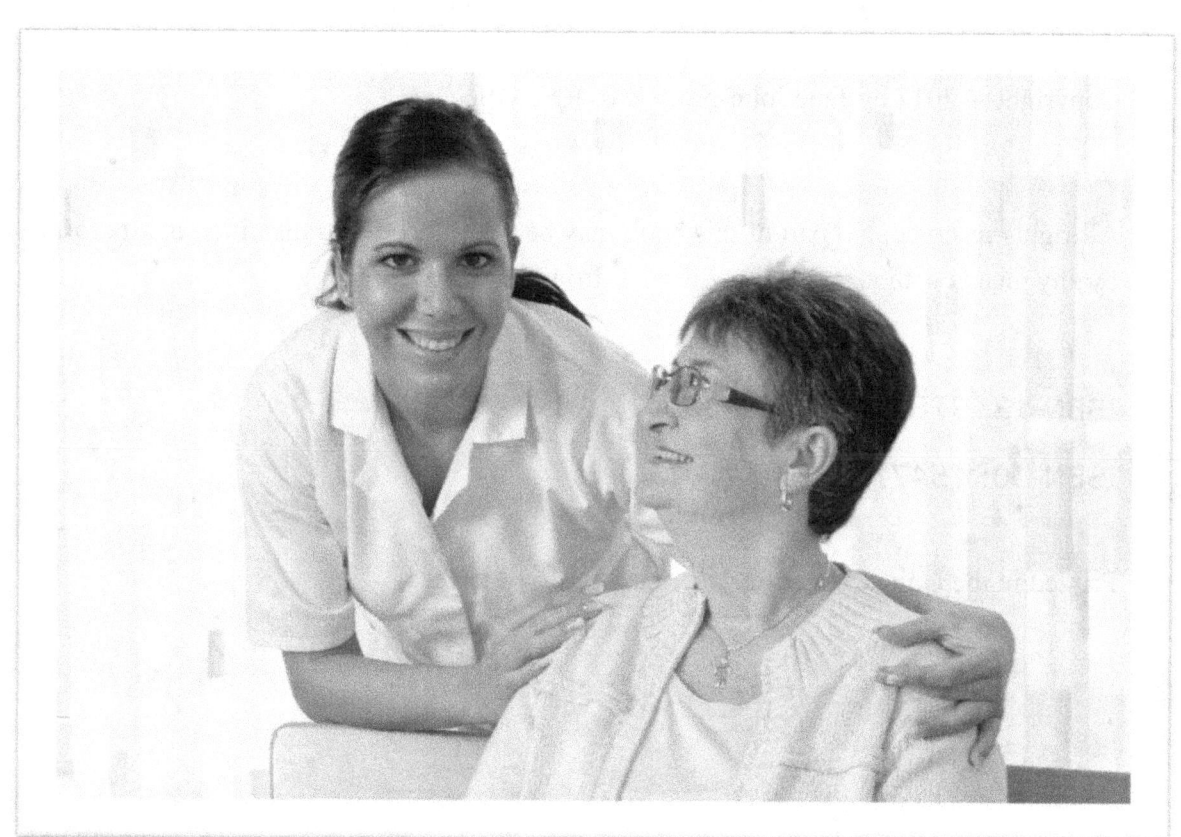

———

Jane John-Nwankwo   CPT, DSD, RN, MSN, PHN

Workbook

Home Health Aide Textbook

Home Care Principles

ISBN-13: 978-1547179503

ISBN-10: 1547179503

Printed in the United States of America.

Have you bought these books?

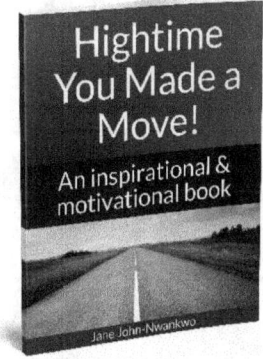 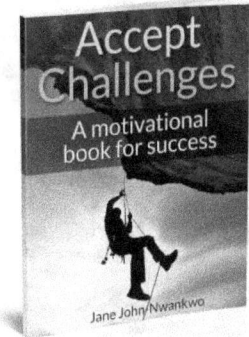 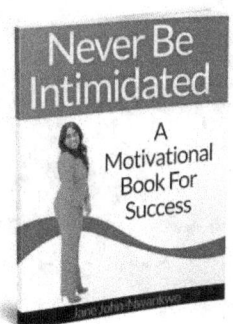

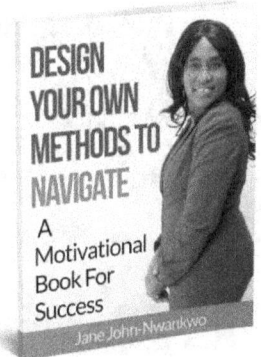 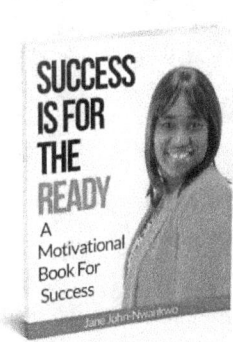 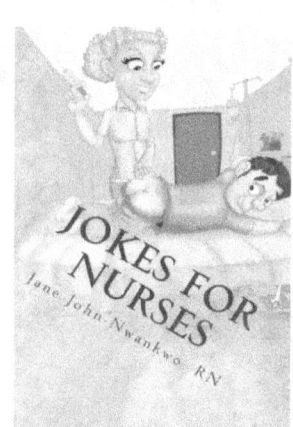

www.janejohn-nwankwo.com

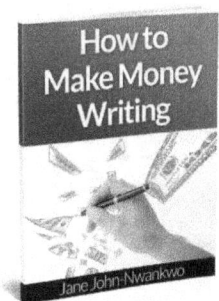 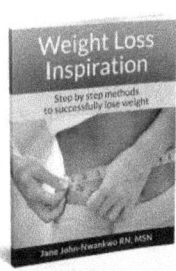 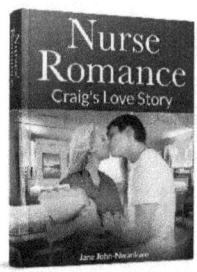 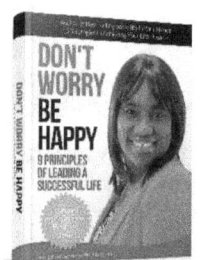

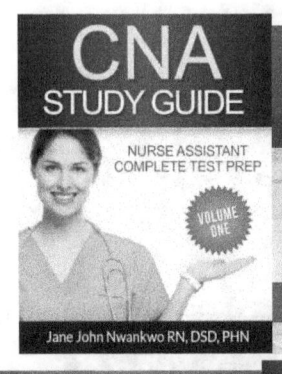
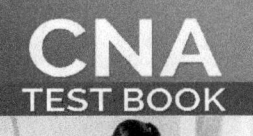
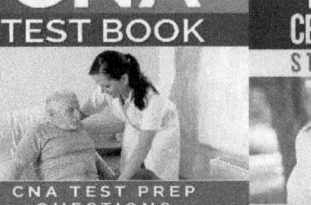
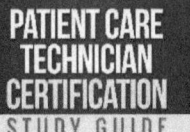
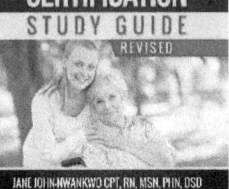
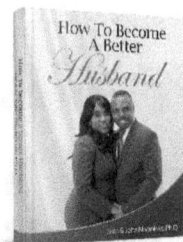
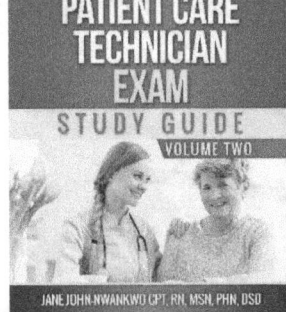
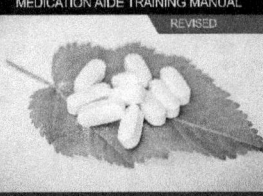
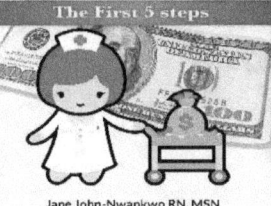
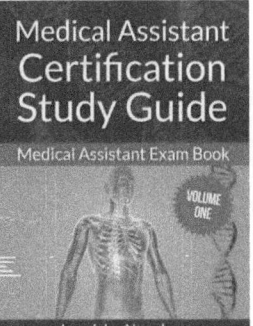
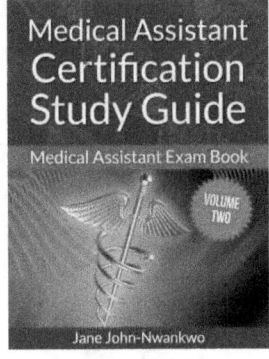
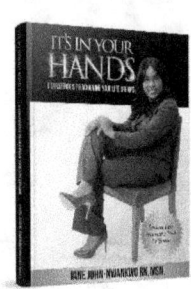
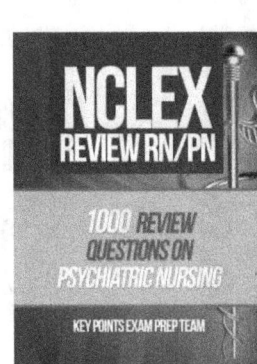
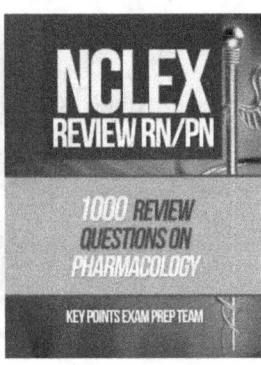

www.janejohn-nwankwo.com

Dedication

To my loving daughter, Jessica Chinyere John-Nwankwo

Table of Contents

Chapter 1

Introduction to the Home Health Agency Roles………..

Chapter 2

Medical and Social needs of Home Care clients……..

Chapter 3

Personal Care Services by the Home Health Aide….....

Chapter 4

Nutrition in Home Care …………………………

Chapter 5

Cleaning Tasks in the Home……………………….......

Chapter 6

Infection Prevention in Home Care ………….……....

Chapter 7

Vital Signs……………………………………… …

Bonus Reading for Caregivers …....................

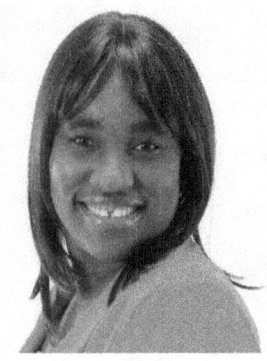

From the author

This workbook accompanies Home Health Aide Textbook which was written out of an inner passion to provide a quality, but concise textbook for Home Health Aides as well as Caregivers. If the reader gains any new knowledge from this book or finds new strength to care for people who require care in their homes, then the purpose of this book would have been achieved.

- Jane John-Nwankwo RN, MSN.

Author, Public speaker,

Educational consultant

support@janejohn-nwankwo.com

www.janejohn-nwankwo.com

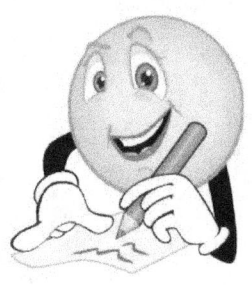

Chapter One

Introduction to the Home Health Agency Role

Outline

1. Introduction

2. State and federal regulations and requirements for HHA certification

3. Purpose and goals of home health care

4. Members of the home health care team

5. Roles and responsibilities of the certified home health aide

6. Common observations and documentation to be done by the HHA

7. Key steps in the communication process and methods of communication

8. Key steps in accommodating communication with clients with hearing or speech disorders.

9. Effective techniques for communication with home health team members

10. Effective communication in learning about clients.

11. Access to community agencies to meet client needs

12. Organizational and time management techniques for a daily work schedule.

13. Conclusion

1. Home Healthcare may consist of which of the following?
   a. Nursing care
   b. Occupational therapy
   c. Speech therapy
   d. Any of the above

2. Which healthcare team member collaborates with doctors to give patients the proper care he/she needs?
   a. Pharmacist
   b. Nurse
   c. Physical therapist
   d. Social worker

3. Which team member is concerned with how disease/illness affects the patient's ability to function normally?
   a. Speech therapist
   b. Physical therapist
   c. Occupational therapist
   d. None of the above

4. Which team member provides emotional and psychological support to the home care team?
   a. Pharmacist
   b. Nurse
   c. Physical therapist
   d. Social worker

5. Which team member helps patients recover and develop his/her skills to communicate?
   a. Speech therapist
   b. Physical therapist
   c. Occupational therapist
   d. None of the above

6. Who directs the home health team?
   a. The home health nurse
   b. The Psychologist
   c. The pharmacist
   d. The social worker

7. What is the role of the HHA?
    a. To provide emotional and psychological support for the team
    b. To provide personal care for the patient
    c. To help the patient gain a higher level of independence
    d. To coordinate the services being provided

8. Which of the following might be included in the responsibilities of the HHA?
    a. Grooming
    b. Changing bed linens
    c. Bathing the patient
    d. All of the above

9. Which of the following should be documented by the HHA?
    a. Headaches
    b. Change of appetite
    c. Joint pain
    d. All of the above

10. Which of the following is not a key in the communication process?
    a. Thought
    b. Creation
    c. Transmission
    d. Reception

11. Which of the following team members has the most contact with the patient?
    a. Nurse
    b. Doctor
    c. Home health aide
    d. Occupational therapist

12. Which of the following statements about the patient's written record is false?
    a. It should be regularly updated by team members
    b. It is one of the most effective techniques of team communication
    c. It should be updated regularly
    d. It is meant to be an urgent form of communication between team members

13. Which of the following is not essential to the HHA's communication?
    a. Clarity of the record
    b. Abbreviating to save space
    c. Confidentiality
    d. Accuracy of the record

14. Which of the following statements is false about home healthcare?
    a. It is unique to the patient's needs
    b. It is more cost effective than hospital care
    c. It is a way to push patients out of the hospital onto other caregivers
    d. It requires a team of professionals for effective care

15. Who writes the prescriptions when a patient is under home healthcare?
    a. The doctor
    b. The nurse
    c. The home health aide
    d. Any of the above

16. Which of the following is true about seeing the patient at home?
    a. The patient usually is uncomfortable about allowing strangers into the house
    b. The nurse can possibly identify environmental factors that contribute to illness
    c. The patient never has to go out for medical care
    d. The home health aide acts in the place of the doctor or nurse

17. Which of the following statements is true?
    a. A home health patient always needs services of nurses, various therapists, and health aides
    b. Patients always fully recover with home healthcare services
    c. The treatment plans may change based on changes noted by the nurse
    d. The RN always makes the final decision for any needed interventions

18. Which of the following is not a way to manage your time?
    a. Prioritize your tasks
    b. Identify your goals
    c. Be a perfectionist
    d. Review your time utilization

19. Which of the following will give you more effective communication with your patient?
    a. Maintain eye contact
    b. Observe body language
    c. Avoid jargon
    d. All of the above

20. Which of the following is not an effective way for the home health team to communicate?
    a. The case conference

b. Written documentation

c. Phone calls

d. Text messages

21. If a client is hard of hearing you may want to:
    a. Speak clearly and loudly
    b. Write communications
    c. Shout
    d. A and B only

22. Which of the following statements about communicating with a hearing impaired patient is false?
    a. You should not assume that you know what the patient is going to say
    b. Never be in a hurry
    c. Shout if necessary
    d. Face the client in case he or she compensates by reading lips

23. Which of the following statements about communicating with patients is false?
    a. Allow the patient to finish his/her sentences
    b. Encourage sign language in patients that are attempting to learn to speak again
    c. Ask yes or no questions
    d. If a patient hears better out of a certain ear attempt to stand by it

24. Which of the following is not something to document in the patient's record?
    a. Weight gain or loss
    b. Type of TV show that the patient watches
    c. Bouts of depression
    d. Loss of range of motion

25. Who can assist with some of the home healthcare tasks?
    a. Certified aides
    b. Family members
    c. Paid companions
    d. All of the above

26. Which of the following tasks is not the responsibility of the home health aide?
    a. Changing linens
    b. Bathing the patient
    c. Assisting with basic exercise
    d. All of the above are responsibilities of the HHA

27. Which of the following about speech therapists is false?
   a. The speech therapist uses a wide range of communication aids and technology
   b. The speech therapist will help the patient fully recover the patient's vocal capabilities
   c. The speech therapist teaches compensatory communication methods for those who have lost the ability to speak
   d. The speech therapist may teach sign language or use of a communication board

28. Which of the following about occupational therapists is false?
   a. The occupational therapist helps patients achieve a higher level of independence
   b. The occupational therapist can help the patient make adjustments to the home and to belongings to improve functionality
   c. The occupational therapist is concerned with how a disease or illness affects a patient's everyday life
   d. The occupational therapist does day to day tasks for the patient

29. When are most skills taught to home health aides?
   a. During college classes
   b. During training
   c. During HHA exams
   d. During hospital orientation

30. What is the job of the physical therapist?
   a. Help increase the patient's mobility and reduce risks of falling
   b. Assist in helping the patient communicate
   c. Bathe the patient and change linens
   d. All of the above

31. Which of the team is available through a 24 hour on call system?
   a. The occupational therapist
   b. The pharmacist
   c. The social worker
   d. The home health aide

32. Which of the following should you not do when writing in the patient's record?
   a. Write clearly
   b. Abbreviate as much as possible
   c. Write in short, concise sentences

d. Write specific observations

33. If you make a mistake in the patient record you should:
    a. Use Whiteout or correction tape
    b. Use on clear line to mark through your mistake
    c. Use a Sharpie to black out your mistake
    d. Throw the paper away and start over

34. Which of the following statements about home healthcare is true?
    a. The outcome of home healthcare depends on one key team member
    b. All patients follow the same healthcare plan
    c. The patient receives all of the same care that he/she would receive at the hospital
    d. One of the most important parts of home healthcare is the documentation

35. Which of the following statements is true?
    a. All home health aides must be certified nationally
    b. All home health aides must take 75 to 200 hours of healthcare classes
    c. Most skills are taught by other healthcare workers during training
    d. All home healthcare offers the same care to each patient

36. Who works with both the physician and the team to coordinate services provided?
    a. The nurse
    b. The home health aide
    c. The occupational therapist
    d. The physical therapist

37. Which person on the team is primarily responsible for ensuring that other team members understand how to administer medication?
    a. The speech therapist
    b. The physical therapist
    c. The pharmacist
    d. The patient's family member

38. Who relays important information about intervention and ancillary services to the physicians?
    a. The occupational therapist
    b. The nurse
    c. The patient
    d. The home health aide

39. Who is the link between formal and informal support services?
   a. The doctor
   b. The nurse
   c. The home health aide
   d. The social worker

40. Who provides personal care for the patient?

a. The home health aide

b. The doctor

c. The social worker

d. The nurse

SAMPLE HOME HEALTH AIDE QUESTIONS

1) ……………..provides assistance to the chronically ill, the elderly, and family caregivers who need relief from the stress of care-giving?

   A) Home health Aids

   B) Pastors

   C) Engineers

   D) Surgeons

2) Agencies pay home health aides from payments they receive from the following payers:

   A) Insurance companies

   B) Health maintenance organizations

   C) Medicare

   D) All of the above

3) The Centre for Medicare and Medicaid services payment system for home care is called the:

A) Home health prospective payment system

B) Pay per charge

C) Service payment

D) Medical payment

4) Clients who need home care are referred by a doctor to a:

A) Hospital

B) Friend

C) Neighbor

D) Home health agency

5) All home health aides are under supervision of one of the following skilled professionals:

A) An engineer

B) A pastor

C) A registered nurse

D) Native medicine

6) All of the following constitute the team of health professionals except:

A) Home health aides

B) Nurses

C) Doctors

D) Engineers

7) ....helps clients learn to compensate for disabilities:

A) A client

B) An occupational therapist

C) Speech language pathologist

D) Registered dietitian

8) A legal term that means someone can be held responsible for harming someone else is referred to as:

    A) Assets

    B) Liability

    C) Action

    D) Discipline

9) A particular method, or way, of doing something is called:

    A) Orientation

    B) A procedure

    C) An activity

    D) Information

10) A professional relationship with a client includes:

    A) Maintaining a negative attitude

    B) Not finishing assignments

    C) Doing only the tasks assigned

    D) None of the above

11) Professionalism means:

    A) Having to do with work or a job

    B) Your life outside your job

    C) Disapproving client's opinion

    D) Keeping late to work

12) ....teaches clients and their families about special diets to improve their health and help them manage their illness:

    A) A medical social worker

    B) A registered dietitian

    C) An occupational therapist

    D) None of the above

13) A professional relationship with an employer does not include of the following:

A) Always being on time

B) Completing assignments efficiently

C) Maintaining a negative attitude

D) Participating in education programs offered

14) Which of the following depicts the meaning of laws?

A) Laws are rules set by the government

B) Laws tell us what we must do

C) Laws help to ensure order and safety

D) All of the above

15) ………………defines the things you are allowed to do and describes how to do them correctly:

A) A plan

B) A liability

C) A procedure

D) A scope of practice

16) Which of the following is not an example of legal and ethical behavior by HHAs?

A) Protecting client's privacy

B) Accepting gifts and tips

C) Being honest at all times

D) Documenting accurately and promptly

17) Clients have the right to:

A) Have access, upon request, to all bills   for service the client has received

B) Receive care of the highest quality

C) Refuse services without fear of reprisal

D) All of the above

18) Unexplained injuries including burns, bruises, and bone injuries can be referred to as:

    A) Mental abuse

    B) Physical abuse

    C) Psychological abuse

    D) Passive neglect

19) You can help protect your client's rights in which of the following ways:

    A) Respect your clients' property

    B) Talk or gossip about a client

    C) Neglect clients in your planning

    D) Enter a client's room without knocking and seeking permission

20) To respect confidentiality means:

    A) To tell the a client's best friend about his friend's health condition

    B) To keep private things secret

    C) To discuss issues about a client with in a family meeting

    D) None of the above

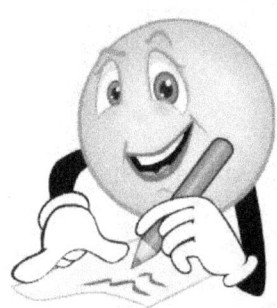

CHAPTER TWO

Medical and social needs of home care clients.

Outline.

1. Introduction

2. Basic physical and emotional needs of clients

3. Recognizing the role of HHA

4. Relating client and family rights to Maslow's hierarchy of needs

5. Culture, lifestyle and life experiences

6. Common reactions to illness/disability

7. Description of basic body functions and changes that should be reported

8. Diseases and disorders common in the healthcare clients

9. Common emotional and spiritual needs

10. Conclusion

1. Which of the following is an example of a patient that might receive home healthcare?
   a. A middle aged double amputee
   b. An elderly person recovering from a heart attack
   c. A child with a mental disability
   d. All of the above

2. Which of the following is a task that the home health aide may assist with?
   a. Bathing
   b. Grooming
   c. Incontinence issues
   d. All of the above

3. Which of the following is not a task that the home health aide may do?
   a. Change complex bandages
   b. Change simple bandages
   c. Assist in serving foods
   d. None of the above

4. Which of the following is not acceptable behavior for the home health aide?
   a. Providing emotional support for the patient
   b. Providing emotional support for the family
   c. Discriminating because of culture or religion
   d. Cooperating with the client and family

5. Which of the following is a physiological need?
   a. Employment
   b. Food
   c. Belonging
   d. Self-esteem

6. Which of the following is considered a safety need?
   a. Belonging
   b. Self-esteem
   c. Protection from germs
   d. Food

7. Which of the following is considered a belonging need?
    a. Support of family and friends
    b. Self-esteem
    c. Protection from germs
    d. Food

8. Which of the following is considered a need for self-esteem?
    a. Respect
    b. Protection from germs
    c. Food
    d. Employment

9. Which of the following is the highest level of Maslow's hierarchy?
    a. Belonging
    b. Physiological needs
    c. Self-actualization
    d. Safety

10. Which of the following levels of Maslow's hierarchy explains that it is important for people to be allowed to make their own decisions?
    a. Safety
    b. Self-actualization
    c. Belonging
    d. Physiological needs

11. Which of the following may affect how the patient's family views the patient's illness?
    a. Maslow's hierarchy
    b. The home health aide
    c. Culture and beliefs
    d. None of the above

12. Which of the following might be offensive to someone of a different culture?
    a. Calling someone honey or sweetie
    b. Touching an image of a god in the patient's house
    c. Picking up an object of sacred value
    d. All of the above

13. What is the definition of culture?
    a. A person's religious beliefs
    b. The sum total of the way of life
    c. A person's thoughts

d. The sum total of the person's actions

14. Which is an effective way of becoming culturally aware?
    a. Identifying cultural prejudice
    b. Identifying fears
    c. Identifying strengths
    d. Identifying weaknesses

15. Once a cultural prejudice is recognized you should:
    a. Tell the client he/she is wrong
    b. Tell the client why you are right
    c. Adjust your behavior to treat the client appropriately
    d. All of the above

16. Which of the following is an example of a cultural belief?
    a. The belief that an illness is punishment because of a person's action
    b. The belief that a medication will help an illness
    c. The belief that a neighborhood is safe
    d. All of the above

17. Which of the following may contribute to a patient refusing to cooperate?
    a. A desire to get better
    b. A desire for help
    c. A negative experience with the healthcare system
    d. A positive experience with the healthcare system

18. Which of the following is an example of a cultural value?
    a. A request for a home health aide
    b. A male family member making all decisions
    c. A request for help dressing
    d. All of the above

19. You have a very superstitious patient that believes in old medicine. However, the old medicine is known to prevent a certain medication from working properly. Which of the following is an appropriate course of action?
    a. Observe the patient's room for signs of old medicine
    b. Document specific comments that you have heard
    c. Notify the RN of your suspicions
    d. All of the above

20. Which of the following may explain a family member's hesitation to administer home care?

a. Excitement about the illness
b. Love
c. Fear of contracting the illness
d. All of the above

21. Which of the following may cause stress to the home health patient and his/her family?
    a. Lack of progress in the patient's condition
    b. Sufficient insurance coverage to pay for treatment
    c. Sufficient time to assist with care
    d. Marked improvement in the patient's condition

22. Which of the following may occur when the patient does not get better or further deteriorates?
    a. The family may become over protective
    b. The Patient may begin to feel grief and anxiety
    c. The family may become hostile
    d. All of the above

23. Which of the following statements is true?
    a. As a home health aide you should only be concerned with the patient's needs
    b. As a home health aide you have authority over the patient
    c. As a home health aide you must assess the needs of the patient and the family
    d. As a home health aide the patient and family must listen to you

24. A family is feeling very burdened with finances and care of a patient. You should:
    a. Explain that it's normal and that they should just deal with it
    b. Dismiss their stress
    c. Refer to the family to resources and/or the social worker
    d. Ignore the problem and continue patient care

25. Which of the following is a sign that the patient may be suffering from stress or depression?
    a. A cheerful smile
    b. Refusal to eat
    c. An interest in a new hobby
    d. Being talkative

26. Which of the following changes in the patient must be reported?
    a. High blood sugar in spite of medication

b. Frequent falls

c. High or low blood pressure

d. All of the above

27. Which disorder is characterized by impaired cognition and loss of memory?
    a. Heart disease
    b. Glaucoma
    c. Influenza
    d. Dementia

28. Which of the following is a sign of incontinence?
    a. Forgetfulness
    b. Loss of bladder control
    c. Frequent falls
    d. Chest pain

29. A patient is feeling pain in hands and knees. Which of the following may explain this pain?
    a. Glaucoma
    b. Incontinence
    c. Arthritis
    d. Heart disease

30. Which of the following is a sign of diabetes?
    a. Sweating
    b. High blood glucose
    c. Blurred vision
    d. All of the above

31. Which of the following is characterized by brittle bones?
    a. Diabetes
    b. Stroke
    c. Osteoporosis
    d. Heart disease

32. Which of the following is true about a patient dealing with terminal illness?
    a. He/she will accept it immediately
    b. He/she will probably go through a grieving process
    c. He/she needs to be left alone
    d. None of the above

33. Which of the following are normal reactions to terminal illness?
    a. Anger
    b. Denial
    c. Depression
    d. All of the above

34. Which of the following statements is true?
    a. The family of the terminally ill will also go through stages of grief
    b. The family of the terminally ill will not feel anger about the patient's illness
    c. It only matters how the patient feels
    d. It is best for the family to bottle their emotions for the sake of the patient

35. Which of the following is a good way to deal with grief?
    a. Bottle up the emotions for the sake of the ill
    b. Speak with a family therapist or counselor
    c. Pretend that everything is okay
    d. Both A and C

36. What is another acceptable way to deal with grief?
    a. Seek religious support
    b. Avoid neighbors and friends
    c. Avoid the ill
    d. Say nothing

37. The home health aide does which of the following for the patient?
    a. Assist with bathing and dressing
    b. Assist with housework
    c. Encourage and support the patient
    d. All of the above

38. Which of the following affects the decisions of the client?
    a. Culture
    b. Beliefs
    c. Experience
    d. All of the above

39. Which of the following is a major cause of stress to clients and family?
    a. Financial issues
    b. A good support network
    c. A good prognosis
    d. B and C only

40. A family turns to its oldest son to make decisions about care for their father. This is an example of:
    a. Grief
    b. Culture
    c. Experience
    d. Feminism

21) ………………..is the process of exchanging information with others:

    A) Looking

    B) Recreation

    C) Communication

    D) Interpretation

22) Always report combative behaviors of clients to your:

    A) Parents

    B) Client's friend

    C) Friend

    D) Supervisor

23) All of the following are some barriers to communication, except:

    A) Client hears and understands you clearly

    B) Client is difficult to understand

    C) Asking why

    D) Client speaking in a different language

24) Which of the following questions would you ask a client for adequate clarifications?

    A) Did you sleep last night?

    B) Did he rape you?

    C) Tell me about your sleep last night

    D) Is exercise good?

25) Reasons for documentation include:

    A) It guarantees clear and complete communication

    B) It provides up-to-date record of the status of a client

C) Documentation protects you and the employer from liability

D) All of the above

26) File an incident report when one of the following incidents occurs:

A) You client performs an exercise

B) Your client falls

C) When a patient is safe

D) When a client lies on the right side of the body

27) The process of removing pathogens or state of being free from pathogens is referred to as:

A) Medical asepsis

B) Plasmodiasis

C) Sepsis

D) Toxoplasmosis

28) …………..is where the pathogen lives and grows:

A) House

B) Ecosystem

C) Landscape

D) Reservoir

29) An uninfected person who could get sick or infected is referred to as a:

A) Portal of entry

B) Causative agent

C) Susceptible host

D) Sepsis

30) If blood or body fluid spills on fabrics such as carpets and clothes:

A) Use alcohol to clean it

B) Use commercial disinfectants to clean it

C) Clean with bleach

D) None of the above

31) ………………..is a federal government agency that issues information to protect the health of individuals and communities:

A) Health firm

B) World health organization

C) The centre for disease control and prevention

D) Individual co-operations

32) One of the following is not included as one of the measures of standard precautions:

A) Clean a client's blood without wearing gloves

B) Wash your hands before putting on gloves

C) Wear gloves if you may come in contact with body fluids

D) Wear a disposable gown that is resistant to body fluid

33)………………..refers to washing hands with water and soap or other detergents that contain an antiseptic agent:

A) Hand antisepsis

B) Hand rinsing

C) Protocols

D) None of the above

34) Equipment that helps protect employees from serious injuries or illnesses resulting from contact with workplace hazards is called:

A) Personal protective equipment

B) Standard precaution

C) Hospital policy

D) Health machineries

35) Personal protective equipment includes the following, except one:

A) Masks

B) Goggles

C) Gowns

D) Needles

36) One of the following is not an airborne disease:

    A) Measles

    B) Tuberculosis

    C) Boil

    D) Chickenpox

37) Droplets can be created by:

    A) Coughing

    B) Sneezing

    C) Laughing

    D) All of the above

38) An example of a droplet disease is the:

    A) Rash

    B) Scabies

    C) Mumps

    D) Constipation

39) MRSA stands for:

    A) Menstrual reluctant stage of Action

    B) Men Rehabilitation system activities

    C) Methicillin-resistant staphylococcus aureas

    D) None of the above

40) Droplet precautions include:

    A) Wearing a face mask during care

    B) Restricting visits from uninfected people

    C) An infected client covering his nose and mouth with a tissue when sneezing

D) All of the above

41) The way the parts of the body works together whenever you move is referred to as:

A) Body mechanics

B) Movement

C) Body structure

D) Matrix

42) When you stand, your weight is centered in:

A) Elbows

B) Your arms

C) Your pelvis

D) Fibula

43) Disorientation means confusion about:

A) Person

B) Place

C) Time

D) All of the above

44) Burns can be caused by one of the following:

A) Cold water

B) Hand shaking

C) Dry heat

D) Waxing floors

45) Employee's responsibilities for infection control include the following:

A) Follow standard precautions

B) Take advantage of the free hepatitis B vaccination

C) Immediately report any exposure you have to infection, or blood

D) All of the above

46) One of the following is not a guideline to guide against fire:

   A) Stay in or near the kitchen when anything is cooking

   B) Discourage careless smoking and smoking in bed

   C) Turn on heaters when no one is home

   D) Do not leave dryer on when you leave the house

47) To ensure travel safety:

   A) Avoid planning your route

   B) Use turn signals

   C) Encourage distractions from friends

   D) Drive without seat belt

48) Factors that raise the risk for falls include:

   A) Clutter

   B) Slippery floors

   C) Poor lighting

   D) All of the above

49) …………..is emergency care given immediately to an injured person?

   A) Exercise

   B) Head stretching

   C) 9111

   D) First aid

50) The first signs of insulin reaction include one of the following:

   A) Pneumonia

   B) Heart failure

   C) Constipation

   D) Nervousness

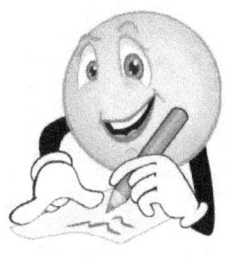

CHAPTER THREE

Personal Care Services by the Home Health Aide

Outline

1. Introduction

2. Steps and guidelines for common personal care

3. Importance of improvising equipment and adapting care activities in the home

4. Personal care delivery at home

5. Examples of equipment that can be used to provide care

6. Benefits of self-care in promoting wellness

7. Key principles of body mechanics

8. How to adapt body mechanics in the home

9. Adaptations that can be made in the home for ambulation and positioning

10. The purpose of passive and active range motion exercise

11. High risk factors for skin breakdown and methods of prevention

12. Stages of pressure ulcers/decubitus ulcers and report observation

13. Types of ostomies and how to empty and change the pouch

14. Emergencies in the home and critical steps to follow

15. The chain of infection to the home care setting

16. Infection control measures to use in the home care setting

17. Role and responsibilities of the HHA in assisting the client to self-administer medications

18. Conclusion

1. Which of the following is an acceptable way to bathe a patient?
   a. Tub bath
   b. Bed bath
   c. Shower bath
   d. All of the above

2. Which of the following must you do before performing a bed bath?
   a. Make sure that the room temperature is warm
   b. Open all of the windows for fresh air
   c. Change the linens
   d. Dress the patient

3. When undressing the patient, which is the last part of the body to have the clothing removed?
   a. The head
   b. The feet
   c. The paralyzed portion
   d. The active portion

4. Which is not a necessary item for a tub bath?
   a. A large bowl or pan
   b. A shower sprayer
   c. Two chairs
   d. Cloths or sponges

5. When bed bathing a patient you should always work from:
   a. Left to right
   b. Top to bottom
   c. Right to left
   d. Bottom to top

6. Which areas of the patient's body should be uncovered?
   a. The paralyzed portion
   b. The feet
   c. The areas that are being cleaned
   d. No areas

7. Proper cleaning of a patient's face is as follows:
   a. Clean the face without soap unless requested, then clean the neck and ears with soap
   b. Clean all areas of the head with soap
   c. Insist that the patient clean his/her own face
   d. Clean the face with soap, then clean the neck and ears without soap

8. When cleaning a patient's chest and abdomen you must be sure to pay attention to the:
   a. Chest
   b. Abdomen
   c. Smooth areas
   d. Skin folds

9. If the patient is physically able to clean his/her perennial area, the home health aide should:
   a. Give the patient the cleaning cloth and look away
   b. Supervise the cleaning to make sure the patient does it right
   c. Have the patient's family member assist with cleaning
   d. Have the patient completely bathe him/her self

10. If the patient cannot clean his/her own perennial area the home health aide should:
    a. Use soap sparingly and clean from front to back
    b. Use a lot of soap and clean from back to front
    c. Not clean it at all
    d. Insist that a family member clean the patient

11. After cleaning the perineal area the home health aide should:
    a. Continue cleaning the rest of the patient
    b. Make sure that the entire perennial area is dry
    c. Have the patient get back into bed
    d. Have the patient dry him/her self

12. When re-dressing a patient you should begin by:
    a. Putting socks on first
    b. Dressing the patient from bottom to top
    c. Dress the paralyzed portions of the body first
    d. Have the patient dress him/her self

13. When lifting a patient you should:
    a. Lift with your back

    b. Lift with your arms

    c. Lift with your legs

    d. Lift with your wrists

14. When lifting a patient your feet should be:
    a. Shoulder width apart
    b. Less than shoulder width apart
    c. Together
    d. More than shoulder width apart

15. Which is a good example of improvising equipment in a patient's home?
    a. Splicing two power cords together with medical tape
    b. Using a plastic chair to assist with bathing
    c. Using medical tape to tape the leg of a broken chair
    d. All of the above

16. Personal care delivery entails which of the following?
    a. Paying attention to safety
    b. Paying attention to comfort
    c. Using available information and skills to deliver care
    d. All of the above

17. Which of the following is true about self-care?
    a. It can lead to good quality of life
    b. It is irrelevant to patient care
    c. It is decided by the family
    d. It is a placebo

18. Which of the following is false about lifting a patient and body mechanics?
    a. The legs should be positions apart
    b. Lift with your legs rather than your back
    c. If you must turn around you should twist rather than move your feet
    d. The lifted object should be close to the body

19. Which of the following is the best way to move a heavy object or person?
    a. Pulling or pushing
    b. Lifting
    c. Asking the doctor for help
    d. Any of the above

20. When reaching for something you should always:
    a. Stand on a swivel chair

b. Stand on tip toes

c. Plant your feet firmly and use a stool if necessary

d. Jump and grab the object

21. Which of the following is not a way to move a patient?
    a. Asking for help
    b. Twisting your body and using your back
    c. Using your legs for leverage
    d. All of the above are good ways to move patients

22. Using different parts of the body to make safe movements and conserve energy and increase efficiency is called:
    a. Precision movement
    b. Body mechanics
    c. Body efficiency
    d. Body dynamics

23. When a patient sits, stands, or moves, it is important to:
    a. Provide physical support to the client
    b. Let the client do it on his/her own
    c. Hold the client's hand
    d. Any of the above

24. Which of the following is considered passive range of motion?
    a. A patient doing arm raises
    b. A patient doing leg lifts
    c. A patient doing chair exercises
    d. A therapist moving and stretching the patient's arm for him/her

25. A patient's physical therapist instructs the patient on how to correctly do exercises. This is an example of:
    a. Active motion
    b. Passive motion
    c. Aerobic instruction
    d. Bodily therapy

26. Which of the following are goals for both active and passive motion?
    a. Build muscle
    b. Build endurance
    c. Prevent atrophy
    d. Increase atrophy

27. Which of the following is a false statement about the skin?
    a. It protects the body
    b. It is a sensory organ
    c. A third of blood circulation occurs in the skin
    d. It is the third largest organ outside of the body

28. Which of the following causes the skin to breakdown?
    a. Sufficient airflow across the skin
    b. Exercise
    c. Friction and moisture
    d. None of the above

29. Which of the following will cause damage to the skin?
    a. Pressure or force on the skin
    b. Lack of padding and elasticity
    c. Loss of sensation in the skin
    d. All of the above

30. Which of the following is common among patients that have a lack of sensation in the skin and reduced mobility?
    a. Pressure sores
    b. Friction burns
    c. Glaucoma
    d. Heat rash

31. Which of the following is known as decubitus?
    a. Injury to the skin or the tissue below the skin from friction and pressure
    b. Injury to the skin or tissue below the skin from excess heat
    c. Injury to the skin or tissue below the skin from excess cold
    d. Injury to the skin or tissue below the skin from a sudden impact

32. Which of the following is true about decubitus?
    a. It is easy to cure
    b. It is not a threat to most home health patients
    c. It can lead to tissue loss, tendon loss, and bone loss
    d. It does not need to be reported

33. What is an ostomy?
    a. An opening on the body where the body has not healed properly
    b. A type of friction sore
    c. A type of decubitus

d. An opening on the body purposely left open after surgery

34. When there is an emergency in the home:
    a. The home health aide should move the patient away from danger if possible
    b. An ambulance should be called
    c. A manager should be notified
    d. All of the above

35. Where might an agent of infection be in a patient's house?
    a. Hands
    b. A surface
    c. Equipment
    d. All of the above

36. Which of the following should be done in order to prevent infection spread?
    a. Wipe things with a dry plain washcloth
    b. Hand washing
    c. Wipe things on your shirt
    d. All of the above

37. Which of the following helps control infection spread?
    a. Using antiseptic wipes on surfaces
    b. Blowing off candy that you have dropped on the floor
    c. Wiping your feet at the door
    d. Drinking rum to kill the germs inside of your body

38. Which of the following is the role of the HHA in helping the patient self-administer medications?
    a. Having the patient remove the medicine caps on his/her own
    b. Checking labels to be sure that you are handing the patient the correct medications
    c. Insisting that the patient retrieve his/her own medication from the medicine cabinet
    d. Giving the patient a handful of pills

39. Which of the following is true about home healthcare?
    a. It is intended to give the client quality healthcare services
    b. It is meant to replace the need for a doctor
    c. It is a luxury service provided to only those who can afford it
    d. It is unnecessary to the patient's recovery

40. Which of the following is true about infections?
    a. They do not pose a health threat to the home health client
    b. They are only a minor concern to the healthcare community
    c. They can be controlled through good hygiene
    d. All of the above

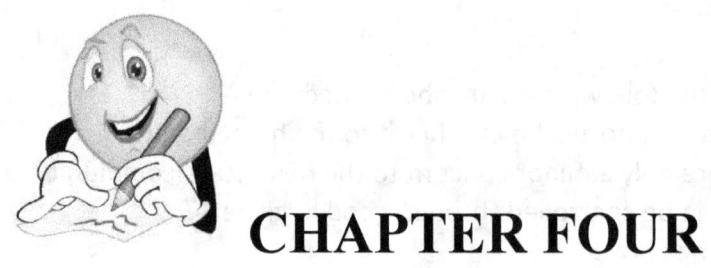

CHAPTER FOUR

Nutrition in Home Care

Outline

1. Introduction

2. Key principles of nutrition

3. Potential nutritional problems

4. Therapeutic diets

5. Safe food handling and storage

6. Adaptations for feeding

7. Fluid balancing

8. Community resources for meeting nutritional needs

9. Conclusion

1. Which of the following will help restore health, strength, and energy to the client?
   a. Exercise
   b. Interesting TV shows
   c. Interacting with family and friends
   d. Good nutrition

2. Which of the following is not a food group?
   a. Carbohydrates
   b. Desserts
   c. Fats
   d. Proteins

3. A good diet:
   a. Helps maintain body weight
   b. Boosts the immune system
   c. Replaces lost vitamins and minerals
   d. All of the above

4. Food is important because:
   a. It makes us feel good
   b. It can be substituted for medication
   c. It gives the body energy
   d. It tastes good

5. Which of the following statements is false?
   a. Food can be replaced with a vitamin or supplement
   b. A wide variety of foods is best
   c. Food gives us energy, vitamins, and minerals
   d. Food is essential for recovery

6. Which of the following may hinder a client from eating properly?
   a. Side effects of medication
   b. Depression
   c. An imbalance diet

d. All of the above

7. Which of the following causes dehydration?
   a. A lack of vitamins
   b. A lack of minerals
   c. A lack of fluids
   d. A lack of fruit and vegetables

8. Which of the following refers to a diet that meets specific physical needs of a client?
   a. The Paleo diet
   b. Therapeutic diets
   c. Vegetarian diets
   d. Brachial diets

9. Which of the following is an example of a therapeutic diet?
   a. Food without sodium
   b. Food low in cholesterol
   c. Low fat foods
   d. All of the above

10. You have a client who recently had jaw surgery. Which of the following diets would be a good choice?
    a. A low sodium diet
    b. A soft food diet
    c. A low sugar diet
    d. A low cholesterol diet

11. Which of the following could lead to further illness for a client?
    a. A well rounded diet
    b. A therapeutic diet
    c. Food that has been improperly handled
    d. Food that has been prepared recently

12. You must help a patient eat. Which of the following should you do?
    a. Feed the client at your own pace
    b. Avoid rushing the client and go at his/her pace
    c. Tell the client to get his/her own food
    d. Give yourself a set time limit for the meal

13. If a patient cannot take food orally, you may have to feed the patient through:
    a. An ostomy

b. A feeding tube
c. A nasal tube
d. The mouth

14. It is important to pay attention to:
    a. The patient's bowel and urinary habits
    b. The patient's TV viewing habits
    c. The patient's card playing habits
    d. None of the above

15. Which of the following can cause fluid loss?
    a. Diarrhea
    b. Water
    c. Nutrition
    d. A feeding tube

16. Which of the following can cause fluid retention?
    a. Renal failure
    b. High sodium
    c. Excess IV fluids
    d. All of the above

17. Which of the following may get out of balance if too much fluids are retained or lost?
    a. Brain cells
    b. Oxygen
    c. Nitrogen
    d. Hormones

18. Fluid balance prevents:
    a. Dementia
    b. Dehydration
    c. Heart disease
    d. Hypoglycemia

19. Which of the following are signs of dehydration?
    a. Constipation
    b. Dryness of the tongue
    c. Sunken eyes
    d. All of the above

20. The fluid record can help detect:
    a. Illness or disease
    b. Depression
    c. Poisoning
    d. MRSA

21. Which of the following must be monitored in order to keep track of hydration?
    a. Sweating
    b. Urine output
    c. Saliva
    d. All of the above

22. Which of the following is important in the nutritional aspect of home healthcare?
    a. Involve the client in decisions as much as possible
    b. Make all decisions based on flavor
    c. Make all decisions based on available ingredients
    d. Make all decisions based on your personal tastes

23. The home health aide should:
    a. Find what works and stick with that
    b. Assess the nutritional needs and adjust periodically
    c. Find what the patient likes and stick with that
    d. Consult a dietician for all decisions

24. Which of the following is false about feeding tubes?
    a. They require accuracy and precision to ensure comfort
    b. They are for ill or post-surgical patients
    c. All feeding tubes are the same for standardization purposes
    d. They must be monitored

25. Which of the following is a best practice for feeding a client?
    a. Feed the client at your own pace and observe silence
    b. Feed the client at his/her pace and engage the client
    c. Feed the client at strict meal times and stick to specific durations
    d. If the patient refuses to eat ignore the patient and do not report it

26. Which of the following is essential in food preparation?
    a. Cook the food to the prescribed temperature in order to kill any germs
    b. If you are busy, leave the food on the counter until you have time to put it away
    c. Save water by using the same cutting board for all types of food without

rinsing

  d. Save time and energy by cooking all foods rare

27. You have a diabetic client. Which of the following should be excluded from the menu?
  a. Broccoli
  b. Chicken
  c. Corn
  d. Cake

28. You have a patient with heart disease. Which of the following should be excluded from the menu?
  a. Boiled chicken
  b. Salad
  c. Salty potato chips
  d. Apples

29. A patient is not happy with the low sodium diet. You should:
  a. Be patient and continue to convince the patient that it is best
  b. Give in and feed the client whatever he/she wants
  c. Hand him/her the salt shaker
  d. Refuse to feed the patient until he/she comes around

30. A patient is showing signs of weight loss. This may be a result of:
  a. Over eating
  b. Eating properly
  c. Under nutrition
  d. All of the above

31. Which of the following is true about proper nutrition?
  a. It can reduce medical costs by reducing illnesses
  b. It is not as important as good medicine
  c. People automatically know what is good for them
  d. It is not essential for strength and energy

32. A patient is on a fixed income and does not always eat lunch in order to save money. Which of the following should you do?
  a. Ignore it because he/she is an adult and knows how to live
  b. Lecture the patient on proper nutrition
  c. Refer him/her to community services that offer reduced meals or deliver meals

d. None of the above

33. Which of the following is not a food group?
    a. Fats
    b. Proteins
    c. Vitamins
    d. Water

34. A patient has not been eating lately. His/her medication was recently changed.
    You suspect that:
    a. The patient is not interested in the therapeutic diet
    b. The patient may be suffering from the side effects of the new medication
    c. There is nothing wrong
    d. The patient is simply tired

35. Which of the following is the best example of a balanced meal?
    a. Chicken, a potato, broccoli, and applesauce
    b. Macaroni and cheese and spaghetti
    c. Hot dogs on a bun and French fries
    d. Hash browns

36. Which of the following is the best example of a balanced meal?
    a. Chili cheese fries
    b. Baked potato with sour cream
    c. A hot pocket
    d. Turkey, sweet potatoes, and broccoli

37. A patient is on a low fat diet. Which of the following should you avoid serving to
    him/her?
    a. Baked chicken
    b. Baked fish
    c. A potato with butter and sour cream
    d. Steamed vegetables

38. A patient is on a soft food diet. Which of the following should you avoid serving
    him/her?
    a. Mashed potatoes
    b. Peas
    c. Applesauce
    d. Whole apples

39. Which of the following is not a low sodium food?
    a. Steamed vegetables
    b. Regular hot dogs
    c. Baked potato with no salt
    d. All of the above are low sodium

40. Which of the following is true about a client's food?

    a. You can eat the leftovers

    b. The client always realizes the value of his/her meal

    c. There can be nutritional problems in spite of paying attention

    d. The client always knows what is best for him/her

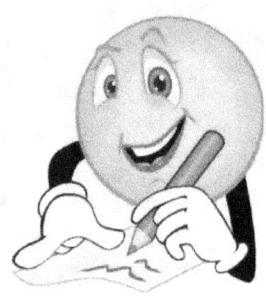

CHAPTER FIVE

Cleaning tasks in home care

Outline

1. Introduction

2. Role of home health aide

3. Principles of safe home environment

4. Procedure, equipment and supplies for house hold tasks

5. Washing and drying dishes

6. Laundering household and personal items

7. Organizing house hold tasks

8. Conclusion

1. Which of the following is important to home safety and avoiding infection?
   a. Making everything look nice
   b. Maintaining cleanliness and order
   c. Pleasant smells for the client
   d. Leaving everything the way you find it

2. You enter a client's home and notice that a chair is in the doorway. You should:
   a. Leave the chair where it is
   b. Close the door so that no one can see the chair
   c. Move the chair so that it does not obstruct mobility
   d. Put the client into the chair

3. Upon meeting a new client you should be sure that:
   a. The client knows how to put out fires
   b. The client can always access the stove
   c. The client has a first aid kit available or first aid supplies
   d. The client is at the top of the stairs

4. Upon meeting a new client you should ensure that:
   a. The client has a working telephone
   b. The client has a working car
   c. The client has a working computer
   d. The client has a working DVD player

5. In order to prevent infection spread, the home health aide can:
   a. Cover his/her mouth when coughing
   b. Wear a mask if the client is sick or coughing
   c. Ensure proper airflow throughout the room
   d. All of the above

6. When changing soiled linens you should:
   a. Throw the soiled linens in with the clean linens
   b. Wrap the soiled linens so that soiling is in the middle
   c. Leave the soiled linens on the bed
   d. All of the above

7. Which of the following should you have for house cleaning?
   a. A maid service
   b. An automatic vacuum

c. A broom

d. An air purifier

8. Which of the following chemicals are basic house cleaning essentials?
    a. Bleach
    b. Water
    c. Old English
    d. All of the above

9. When should you wash your hands?
    a. Before entering the client's house
    b. Before and after each task
    c. After leaving the client's house
    d. Halfway through your visit

10. When handling infectious materials and soiled linens you should:
    a. Spray with Lysol
    b. Spray with bleach
    c. Wear gloves
    d. Wear a hat

11. When cleaning the bathroom you should:
    a. Clean the toilet first then clean the rest of the bathroom with the same rag
    b. Clean the toilet with a disposable cleaning cloth and the rest of the bathroom with a rag
    c. Clean the whole room with Lysol
    d. Let the automatic toilet cleaner do all of the work

12. When cleaning the kitchen you should:
    a. Clean from top to bottom
    b. Clean from bottom to top
    c. Clean with Old English
    d. Clean from left to right

13. The trash should be:
    a. Taken out when full
    b. Taken out when it smells bad
    c. Taken out when it contains infectious materials
    d. Taken out daily

14. The bathroom should be cleaned:
    a. From left to right

b. From bottom to top

c. From top to bottom

d. From right to left

15. When cleaning the floor you should:
    a. Sweep first
    b. Clean the floor after the rest of the room
    c. Dry the floor last
    d. All of the above

16. When washing dishes you should:
    a. Wash the dirtiest items first
    b. Wash with water only
    c. Place everything in the sink together then wash
    d. Use plenty of water and soap

17. When drying dishes you should:
    a. Wipe off with your sleeve
    b. Allow to drip dry, then dry with a clean cloth
    c. Place into the dryer
    d. All of the above

18. If utensils are sterilized you should:
    a. Put them back with other unsterilized utensils
    b. Let them soak in the water extra
    c. Steam the utensils for at least twenty minutes
    d. Disinfect them with a Lysol wipe

19. When doing a client's laundry:
    a. Ask for instructions on using the washer
    b. Sort the clothes by type and color
    c. Empty the pockets
    d. All of the above

20. When drying laundry:
    a. Have the patient dry clothes him/her self
    b. Air dry the clothes that cannot be put into the dryer
    c. Put the clothes back into the washer
    d. All of the above

21. When doing household tasks:
    a. Do everything the client asks

b. Sort and prioritize the tasks
c. Do only the tasks that you want to do
d. Do only the tasks that the family requests

22. When there are too many tasks to handle:
    a. Skip your least favorite tasks
    b. Do a quick, half-hearted job
    c. Request assistance
    d. Any of the above

23. You notice a spill on the kitchen counter. You should:
    a. Leave it until kitchen cleaning day
    b. Wipe up spills daily
    c. Have the client wipe it up
    d. Do nothing

24. Which of the following is essential to household cleaning?
    a. An extendable duster
    b. A mop
    c. Vinegar and newspaper
    d. All of the above are essential

25. In the bathroom, which should be cleaned last?
    a. The toilet
    b. The shower
    c. The sink
    d. The floor

26. When should you wear gloves?
    a. When handling clean utensils
    b. When handling soiled linens and clothes
    c. When handling cleaning chemicals
    d. When handling clean linens and clothes

27. When a patient is coughing or has the flu you should:
    a. Reschedule your visit
    b. Stand closer so that the patient doesn't strain to talk
    c. Wear a mask and don't stand too close
    d. None of the above

28. If a patient falls in the hallway frequently:
    a. You should encourage the patient to walk faster

b. You should discourage the patient from moving
c. You should encourage installation of hand rails
d. You should encourage extra padding in the carpet

29. You walk in and notice a pair of shoes on the floor by the patient's bed. You should:
    a. Encourage the patient to move the shoes
    b. Encourage the patient to wear the shoes
    c. Move the shoes and tell the patient where you are putting them
    d. None of the above

30. Which of the following can prevent accidents?
    a. Helping the patient move about the house
    b. Assist the patient in taking medications
    c. Assisting the patient at meals
    d. All of the above

31. Which of the following is not a risk that home health aides must worry about?
    a. The risk of burns
    b. The risk of choking
    c. The risk of misusing medications
    d. The risk of burglary

32. You enter a client's home and notice glass on the floor. You should:
    a. Let the client know that it's there
    b. Sweep up the glass
    c. Notify the case manager
    d. Refer the client to a cleaning service

33. If the soiled linens and the clean linens are in the same room you must:
    a. Keep the linens separate
    b. Do not keep them in the same room
    c. Install air purification
    d. Burn the dirty linens

34. It is a good idea to:
    a. Leave the cleaning chemicals by the patient's bedside in case he/she needs it
    b. Put chemicals into easy to open bottles
    c. Lock the cleaning chemicals safely away in a cabinet
    d. None of the above

35. If the client does not own a vacuum:
    a. Ignore any carpets
    b. Sweep the carpets with a broom
    c. Mop the carpets
    d. Have the carpets replaced

36. Before sweeping or vacuuming:
    a. Mop the floor
    b. Throw away any large trash from the floor
    c. Disinfect with Lysol
    d. Clean the bathroom

37. When disinfecting utensils:
    a. Place the glass in the bottom of the pot
    b. Place the glass in the top of the pot
    c. Wipe everything with a cloth then put away
    d. Do nothing

38. When laundering clothes and linens:
    a. Wash your hands during the process
    b. Wash the clothes and linens by hand
    c. Wear gloves
    d. All of the above

39. Which of the following is true?
    a. Your tasks must be done on every visit
    b. Your tasks can be done however you wish
    c. Some tasks can be done weekly or monthly depending on the task
    d. The importance of the tasks is up to you

40. After arranging and prioritizing tasks:
    a. Complete all tasks
    b. Remove unnecessary tasks
    c. Complete the tasks you feel like doing
    d. Have the client do the tasks

51) All human beings have the same basic physical needs which include:

A) Food and water

B) Activity

C) Sleep and rest

D) All of the above

52) One of the following is not a psychosocial need:

A) Love and affection

B) Shelter

C) Security

D) Self esteem

53) A system of learned behaviors, practiced by a group of people that are considered to be the tradition of that people is called:

A) Actualization

B) Tribe

C) Culture

D) Precision

54) ………..is the name for the condition in which all of the body's systems are their best?

A) Homeostasis

B) Metabolism

C) Peristalsis

D) Arthritis

55) Which of the following is not a system of the body?

A) Endocrine system

B) Diving system

C) Urinary system

D) Nervous system

56) When the outside temperature is too high, the blood vessels:

A) Constrict

B) Becomes excited

C) Dilate

D) Shortens

57) Which of the following gives the body shape and structure?

A) Apocrine and eccrine structures

B) Veins

C) Arteries

D) Bones and ligaments

58) The nervous system controls and coordinates all body functions.

A) True

B) False

59) The taking-in (breathing in) of oxygen by the body is referred to as:

A) Inspiration

B) Expiration

C) Purification

D) Exchange

60) The largest system organ and the system in the body are the:

A) Mouth

B) Skin

C) Esophagus

D) The small intestine

61) One of the following is a common musculoskeletal system disorder?

A) Nephrotic syndrome

B) Histoplasmosis

C) Pneumonia

D) Osteoporosis

62) The digestive system is also called:

A) Respiratory system

B) Gastro-intestinal Tract

C) Metabolic system

D) Nervous system

63) The two major functions of gastrointestinal system are:

A) Digestion and elimination

B) Digestion and locomotion

C) Elimination and respiration

D) None of the above

64) Endocrine glands secrete:

A) Hormones

B) Enzymes

C) Lipase

D) Amylase

65) The sex cells are formed in the male and female sex glands called the:

A) Gonads

B) Androgens

C) Estrogens

D) Lymphatic

66) At age 1-3 toddlers learn to:

A) Choose education

B) Speak

C) Prepare for retirement

D) Develop language skills and vocabularies

67) ....is a disease or condition that will eventually cause death?

A) A recuperating disease

B) An acute condition

C) Reproductive system

D) A terminal disease

68) The term for the special care a dying person needs is called?

A) Skin care

B) Hospice care

C) Recuperation

D) Advancement stage

69) Which of the following is not included in the normal changes of aging?

A) Incontinence

B) Immunity weakens

C) Appetite decreases

D) Short-term memory loss occurs

70) Common disorders found in infancy period include:

A) Prematurity

B) Low birth weight

C) Sudden infant death syndrome

D) All of the above

71) Which of the following are the basic body positions?

A) Supine

B) Lateral

C) Prone

D) All of the above

72) One of the most important things to consider when transferring a client to a chair or a bed is:

A) Safety

B) Nutrition

C) The Family

D) Finance

73) Contractures are generally caused by:

A) Exercise

B) Driving

C) Locomotion

D) Immobility

74) Pulling a client across sheets can cause:

A) Fluid retention

B) Shearing

C) Spinal cord damage

D) None of the above

75) …………..is a device, such as splint or a brace, which helps support and align a limb and improve its functioning?

A) Leaning table

B) An orthotic device

C) Hand role

D) Head pillows

76) Hygiene and grooming activities, as well as dressing, eating and toileting are called?

      A) Activities of daily living

      B) Recreational activities

      C) Indoor activities

      D) Unhealthy life styles

77) Oral care should be performed at least:

      A) Once a day

      B) At bed time

      C) Twice a day

      D) None of the above

78) ……………is the inhalation of food, fluid or foreign material into the lungs?

      A) Expiration

      B) Inspiration

      C) Aspiration

      D) Asphyxia

79) Moving a body part towards the midline of the body is referred to as:

      A) Supination

      B) Phonation

      C) Rotation

      D) Adduction

80) One of the following is not done if a client starts to fall during a transfer?

      A) Try to reverse or stop a fall

      B) Widen your stance

      C) Call for help if a family member is around

      D) Do not try to reverse or stop a fall

81).................is the impairment of physical or mental functions:

    A) A disability

    B) Burn

    C) Neuralgia

    D) Heart failure

82) A fallacy is:

    A) An opinion

    B) Truth

    C) Being sure

    D) A false belief

83) Which of the following can cause mental illness or make it worse?

    A) Heredity

    B) Stress

    C) Environmental factors

    D) All of the above

84) Sadness is the only one symptom of:

    A) Happiness

    B) Depression

    C) Hopefulness

    D) Excitement

85) Arthritis causes:

    A) Dementia

    B) Tuberculosis

    C) Constipation

    D) Stiffness and pain

86) In diabetes mellitus, the pancreas does not produce enough:

A) Estrogen

B) Prolactin

C) Insulin

D) Progesterone

87) Type 2 diabetes can also be referred to as:

A) Adult-onset diabetes

B) Electrically-charged insufficiency

C) Childbearing diabetes

D) All of the above

88) Paralysis on one side of the body is called:

A) Hemiplegia

B) Aphasia

C) Quadriplegia

D) Dysphagia

89) Risk factors for cancer include the following, except:

A) Poor nutrition

B) Water

C) Radiation

D) Tobacco use

90) A brain disorder that affects a person's ability to think and communicate clearly is called:

A) Anemia

B) AIDS

C) Paresis

D) Schizophrenia

91) Which of the following practices are accepted during housekeeping?

A) Be organized when performing tasks

B) Main a safe environment

C) Familiarize yourself with the household's cleaning materials

D) All of the above

92) Cleaning of the kitchen should be done:

A) Once a day

B) At night only

C) After every use

D) Once in a week

93) Which of the following is an example of a detergent?

A) Soap

B) Iodine

C) Kerosene

D) Anion

94) The process of giving special treatment to items that have heavy soil, spots,, and stains before washing them is called:

A) Retreating

B) Escalation

C) Retouching

D) Pretreating

95) Which of the following would be the reason for changing bed linens?

A) The sheets are wrinkled, making a client uncomfortable

B) The linen was used by another client

C) The linen is damp or unclean

D) All of the above

96) The process by which nutrients are broken down to be used by the body for energy and other needs is referred to as:

A) Reproduction

B) Metabolism

C) Excitation

D) Lyses

97) There are …………..nutrients needed by the body for growth and development:

A) Three

B) Two

C) Six

D) Four

98) Foods high in sodium include the following, except:

A) Bacon

B) Ham

C) Sausage

D) Orange

99) The state of being frightened, excited, confused, in danger or irritated is referred to as:

A) Stress

B) Joy

C) Mood change

D) None of the above

100)…………..occurs when a person does not have enough fluid in his body?

A) Dehydration

B) Fluid overload

C) Crackles in the lungs

D) Water toxicity

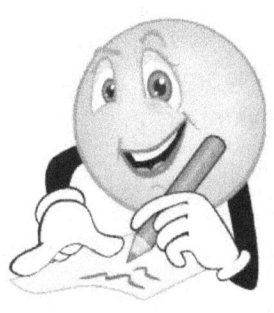

CHAPTER SIX

Prevention of Infection in Home Health Care

Outline

Introduction

Types of infections encountered in home care

Modes of transmission and ways of prevention

Personal Protective Equipment (PPE) in home health care

Conclusion

1. Which of the following contributes to infection existing in the home?
    a. The level of pathogen existence in the home is not terribly uniform
    b. The disinfectants in homes are not as potent
    c. Some clients do not have brooms
    d. Some clients do not have mops

2. Which of the following is a common cause of home infection?
    a. Failure to obey medical advice
    b. Failure to take medicine
    c. Contact with a contaminated object or organism
    d. Contact with children

3. Which of the following is a false statement?
    a. Pathogens in the patient's home are harmless
    b. Hand washing can help reduce contamination
    c. Cleanliness is important to reduce infection
    d. Wearing gloves can help reduce infection

4. Which of the following increases the patient's susceptibility to pathogens in the home?
    a. Super germs in the home
    b. Failure to use bleach in the house
    c. A weakened immune system
    d. A dirty bathroom

5. A patient's family regularly leaves dirty dishes in the sink. You should:
    a. Tell the family that this can increase risk of infection
    b. Ignore the problem
    c. Have the patient do the dishes
    d. Stop washing dishes since no one else is doing it

6. As a home health aide you must:
    a. Be totally responsible for the cleanliness of the house
    b. Offer advice to the family on how to reduce risk of infection
    c. Keep the house sterile
    d. All of the above

7. You walk into a patient's home and notice that the family does not wear gloves when handling soiled linens. You should:

a. Explain the importance of gloves
b. Ignore what is happening
c. Tell the family not to touch the patient
d. Change the linens and clothing yourself only on your visits

8. Which of the following is not an example of infection danger?
a. Decubitus
b. Soiled linens
c. Sick family members
d. Dirty dishes

9. Because the patient's home is not subject to the same regulations as a hospital:
a. The home may have more pathogens
b. The home health aide must teach the client and the family how to reduce infection risk
c. The client may not realize he/she is at risk for infection
d. All of the above

10. Which of the following will reduce risk of infection in the client's home?
a. Wiping everything on your sleeve
b. Opening windows
c. Good cleaning practices
d. None of the above

11. Which of the following will reduce risk of infection in the client's home?
a. Good hygiene for the client
b. Only cleaning when you feel like it
c. Leaving infection control to the family
d. All of the above

12. Which of the following will help the client fight infection?
a. Staying in the hospital
b. Medication
c. Good nutrition
d. Exposing clients to germs to build immunity

13. Which of the following statements is true?
a. Homes have different needs and infection risks than hospitals
b. Gloves help prevent infection spread
c. You should wash your hands before and after each task
d. All of the above

14. You walk into a patient's house and notice a strong odor coming from the garbage can. You should:
    a. Take out the trash and point out that old trash is an infection risk
    b. Leave it for someone else
    c. Light a candle
    d. Spray Lysol

15. Which of the following statements is false?
    a. Families know how to control infections in their own homes
    b. Homes have the same pathogens as hospitals
    c. Infection control methods in hospitals work just the same for houses
    d. All statements are false

16. Which of the following statements is true?
    a. Some infection control methods used in hospitals can also be applied to homes
    b. Gloves and hand washing are a key defense in spreading disease
    c. Wearing masks is an effective form of preventing germ spread
    d. All above statements are true

17. Who should spread knowledge of how to prevent infections?
    a. The client
    b. The home health aide
    c. The client's family
    d. Friends

18. Which of the following creates a high risk for spreading infection?
    a. The client's toilet
    b. Soiled linens
    c. The client's doorbell
    d. The client's family

19. It is important to attempt to:
    a. Reduce the pathogens that the client is exposed to
    b. Inspect the client's house with white glove
    c. Mind your own business
    d. Try not to insult the client with comments on cleanliness

20. Which of the following is an example of an infection risk?
    a. Cleaning the floor with a mop
    b. Washing laundry while wearing gloves
    c. Forgetting to wear gloves when changing a diaper

d. Dustin the ceiling fan

21. If you are visiting a client and you are coughing you should:
    a. Cough into your sleeve
    b. Wear a mask
    c. Stand back from the patient
    d. Any of the above

22. Clients are at risk from:
    a. Pathogens existing inside the house
    b. Pathogens that may come in from the outside
    c. A weakened immune system
    d. All of the above

23. Which of the following hospital methods can be introduced to reduce risk of home infection?
    a. Sterilization of all equipment and tools
    b. Negative pressure rooms for isolation
    c. Use of masks and gloves
    d. Sterile rooms

24. Which of the following hospital methods cannot be used in a home health situation for reducing infection risk?
    a. Limiting contact with people from outside the home (isolation)
    b. Use of gowns, shields, and masks by caregivers and visitors
    c. Keeping a room sterile
    d. Hand washing and use of disinfectant

25. Which of the following statements is true?
    a. Hospitals are no longer the top choice for medical care
    b. Home healthcare is a fast growing field
    c. Home health offers the exact same care as a hospital
    d. Every patient is a good candidate for home healthcare

26. In order to best fight infection you should:
    a. Wash your work clothes at the end of each work day
    b. Shower at the end of each work day
    c. Attempt to consume a healthy diet
    d. All of the above

27. Which of the following statements is true?
    a. It is important to educate the client and his/her family on best infection

control practices
b. The family and client will learn all necessary infection control methods by observation
c. It is not important to discuss infection control with the client
d. It is not important to point out possible methods of infection to the family

28. It is important to pay attention to:
    a. All potential causes of infection
    b. Only the main causes of infection
    c. Only your favorite two causes of infection
    d. None of the above

29. Which of the following statements is false?
    a. Clients often think that their houses are clean or clean enough
    b. A light cleaning is enough to kill pathogens and stop infection spread
    c. The home health aide may notice methods of infection that the family did not notice
    d. The home health aide must be aware of all potential infection risks in order to minimize them

30. When washing your hands you should:
    a. Use bleach
    b. Use warm water and soap
    c. Use only water
    d. There is no need to wash hands

31. In order to best help the client and the family the home health aide must:
    a. Be observant and take note of bad practices around the house, then discuss them
    b. Allow the family and client to choose which methods should be followed
    c. Avoid insulting the cleanliness of the home
    d. Do all of the disinfecting for the week and hope it stays clean

32. You notice that a family member is changing a catheter on your client without wearing gloves. You should:
    a. Mind your own business
    b. Shout at the family member
    c. Discuss the importance of gloves
    d. Any of the above are acceptable

33. A client has the flu. You should:
    a. Wash your hands often

b. Wear gloves

c. Wear a mask

d. All of the above

34. Which of the following is not the result of a pathogen?
    a. Staph Aureus
    b. Influenza
    c. Decubitus
    d. Pink Eye

35. A patient has a rash. You should:
    a. Not treat the patient
    b. Wear gloves
    c. Wear a face shield
    d. Cover it with a bandage

36. A patient soils his/her linens. You should:
    a. Wait until the next scheduled linen change to act
    b. Change the linens while wearing gloves
    c. Notify the client's family to handle it
    d. None of the above

37. You cannot eradicate all pathogens in a client's home. However you can:
    a. Encourage good hygiene
    b. Encourage good housekeeping
    c. Teach the client best practices in infection control
    d. All of the above

38. Since a client's home is full of pathogens:
    a. You should discourage use of home health services
    b. You should encourage the client to stay in the hospital
    c. You should teach the client and family best practices
    d. You should encourage the client to join a nursing home

39. When should you wash your hands?
    a. Before and after a task
    b. Only if your hand is dirty
    c. Only if you have sneezed or coughed
    d. Only if your hands smell dirty

It is up to the home health aide to:

a. Offer insights and guidance about pathogens

b. Ensure that the patient does not get sick

c. Make the family care about pathogens

d. All of the above

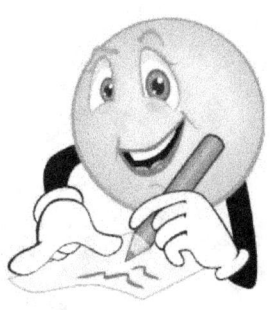

Chapter 7

Vital Signs

Vital signs can reflect the functions of three body processes necessary for life:

Body temperature

Respiration

Heart function

The four vital signs of body function are:

Temperature

Pulse

Respiration

Blood pressure

Chapter Seven

1. What are the four vital signs of the body function?
    A) Temperature, Pulse, Respiration, Digestion.
    B) Temperature, Pulse, Respiration, Blood Pressure.
    C) Temperature, Pulse, Agility, digestion
    D) None of the above.

2. _____ is a balance between heat production and heat loss in conjunction with each other, maintained and regulated by hypothalamus.
    A) Body humidity
    B) Body temperature
    C) Physical balance
    D) Heat balance

3. _____ are used to measure temperature using the Fahrenheit and Centigrade or Celsius scale.
    A) Thermometers
    B) Analog meters
    C) Heat measurers
    D) None of the above.

4. Which of the following is not a temperature measurement site?
    A) The axilla
    B) Tympanic membrane
    C) Mouth
    D) None of the above.

5. Choose the normal temperature range for the oral site.
    A) 98.6 F to 100.5 F
    B) 97.6 F to 99.6 F
    C) 96.6 F to 98.6 F
    D) 95.6 F to 97.6 F

6. Which is the term used to describe the absence of fever?
   A) Febrile
   B) Agile
   C) Afebrile
   D) Able

7. Which of the following is not a type of fever?
   A) Intermittent
   B) Remittent
   C) Continuous
   D) Resilient

8. The fever that remains constant above the baseline and do not fluctuate is called
   _____.
   A) Intermittent
   B) Resilient
   C) Continuous
   D) None of the above.

9. Fluctuating fever that returns to or below baseline then rises again is called as
   _____ fever.
   A) Intermittent
   B) Resilient
   C) Remittent
   D) Continuous

10. On observing the body temperature of a patient you found that the temperature remains elevated and fluctuating. It does not return to base line temperature. What will be your inference?
    A) The patient is suffering from remittent fever and needs treatment.
    B) The patient is suffering from intermittent fever and needs some special treatment.
    C) The patient is agile and can take care of his/her own.
    D) None of the above.

11. _____ is the most common method of measurement.

A) Axillary temperature

B) Oral temperature

C) Tympanic membrane temperature

D) Rectal temperature

12. Oral temperature will not be taken from which of the following patients?
    A) Infants and children less than six years old.
    B) Patients who are receiving oxygen.
    C) Patients who has had surgery.
    D) All the above.

13. Wait for _____ minutes to take the oral temperature in patients who have just finished eating, drinking, or smoking.
    A) 10
    B) 20
    C) 30
    D) 60

14. When taking the temperature, leave the thermometer in the patient's mouth for _____ minutes.
    A) 3 – 5
    B) 10 – 15
    C) 7 – 10
    D) 20

15. _____ temperature is taken when oral temperature is not feasible.
    A) Tympanic membrane
    B) Axillary
    C) Rectal
    D) None of the above.

16. Rectal temperature can be taken for _____.
    A) A patient with heart disease.
    B) A patient with rectal disease.
    C) A patient aged thirty years.
    D) A patient with diarrhoea.

17. _____ is the least accurate measurement.
   A) Oral temperature
   B) Axillary temperature
   C) Rectal temperature
   D) None of the above.

18. Why tympanic temperature is useful for children and confused patients?
   A) Because of the speed of operation of the tympanic thermometer.
   B) Because of the size of the thermometer used.
   C) Because of the attracting appearance of thermometer that do not make the children feel bad.
   D) None of the above.

19. While taking the axillary temperature, the thermometer should be kept in place for _____ minutes.
   A) 5 – 10
   B) 10 – 15
   C) 3 – 5
   D) 20

20. Tympanic temperature measurement cannot be used for whom?
   A) Patients with ear disorder.
   B) Patients with ear drainage.
   C) Either A or B.
   D) Children.

21. The normal adult pulse rate ranges between _____ beats per minute.
   A) 60 and 100
   B) 80 and 100
   C) 80 and 120
   D) 50 and 80

22. Which is the most commonly used site for taking pulse?
   A) Radial artery found in the wrist.
   B) Vertebral vein.

C) Pulmonary artery.

D) Internal carotid artery.

23. The _____ is a more accurate measurement of the heart rate and it is taken over the apex of the heart by auscultation using the stethoscope.

A) Radial artery pulse

B) Apical pulse

C) Carotid pulse

D) Femoral pulse

24. Pulse is taken over the apex of the heart by auscultation using the stethoscope for _____.

A) Patients with irregular heart rate.

B) Infants and small children.

C) Both A and B.

D) All the patients.

25. When measuring respiration, which of the following characteristics will be considered?

A) Rate of respiration

B) Rhythm of respiration

C) Depth of respiration

D) All the above.

26. _____ is the number of respirations per minute.

A) Rate

B) Rhythm

C) Depth

D) None of the above

27. Which of the following is not a respiration rate abnormality?

A) Apnea

B) Tachypnea

C) Bradypnea

D) Cheyne stokes

28. _____ is a regular pattern of irregular breathing rate.

A) Cheyne-Stokes

B) Apnea

C) Orthopnea

D) Bradypnea

29. The difficulty or inability to breath unless in an upright position is called as
_____.

A) Cheyne-Stokes

B) Apnea

C) Orthopnea

D) Bradypnea

30. What is Hyperpnea?

A) A state in which there is an increased amount of air entering the lungs.

B) An abnormal increase in the depth and rate of breathing.

C) A state in which reduced amount of air enters the lungs resulting in decreased oxygen level and increased carbon dioxide level in blood.

D) None of the above.

31. _____ is a state in which reduced amount of air enters the lungs resulting in decreased oxygen level and increased carbon dioxide level in blood.

A) Hypoventilation

B) Hyperpnea

C) Hyperventilation

D) None of the above.

32. _____ is a state in which there is an increased amount of air entering the lungs.

A) Hypoventilation

B) Hyperpnea

C) Bradypnea

D) Hyperventilation

33. _____ refers to the amount of air that is inspired and expired during each respiration.

A) Rate of respiration

B) Rhythm of respiration

C) Depth of respiration

D) None of the above.

34. Which of the following is not an abnormality regarding depth of respiration?

A) Orthopnea

B) Hyperventilation

C) Hypoventilation

D) Hyperpnea

35. The inflatable bag is centred over the _____ artery with the lower border about 2.5cm above the antecubital crease.

A) Vertebral

B) Brachial

C) Right coronary

D) External carotid

36. If the brachial artery is far below the heart level the blood pressure will appear _____.

A) Same as the value which appears when the brachial artery is far above the heart level.

B) Falsely high

C) Falsely low

D) None of the above.

37. Which of the following cannot be considered as the common error in the blood pressure measurements?

A) Improper cuff size.

B) The arm is not at heart level.

C) Cuff is not completely deflated before use.

D) None of the above.

38. Rapid deflation of cuff will lead to _____.

A) Overestimation of systolic and diastolic pressure.

B) Underestimation of systolic and diastolic pressure.

C) Underestimation of the systolic and overestimation of the diastolic pressure.

D) Underestimation of the diastolic and overestimation of the systolic pressure.

39. Which of the following is true regarding anthropometric measurements?
    A) The term anthropometric refers to comparative measurements of the body.
    B) Anthropometric measurements require precise measuring techniques to be valid.
    C) They are used as indicators of the state of health and well-being of the patient and are often included in the initial measurement of vital signs.
    D) All the above.

40. Which of the following is not an anthropometric measurement?
    A) Height
    B) Weight
    C) Body mass index
    D) None of the above.

Answer Key

Chapter One

1. D
2. B
3. C
4. D
5. A
6. A
7. B
8. D
9. D
10. A
11. C
12. D
13. B
14. C
15. A
16. B
17. C
18. C
19. D
20. D
21. D
22. C
23. B
24. B
25. D
26. D
27. B
28. D
29. B

30. A
31. C
32. B
33. C
34. D
35. C
36. A
37. C
38. B
39. D
40. A

Chapter Two

41. D
42. D
43. A
44. C
45. B
46. C
47. A
48. A
49. C
50. B
51. C
52. D
53. B
54. A
55. C
56. A
57. C
58. B
59. D
60. C
61. A
62. D
63. C
64. C
65. B
66. D
67. D
68. B

69. C
70. D
71. C
72. B
73. D
74. A
75. B
76. A
77. D
78. D
79. A
80. B

Chapter Three

1. D
2. A
3. C
4. B
5. B
6. C
7. A
8. D
9. A
10. A
11. B
12. C
13. C
14. D
15. B
16. D
17. A
18. C
19. A
20. C
21. B
22. B
23. A
24. D
25. A
26. C

27. D
28. C
29. D
30. A
31. A
32. C
33. D
34. D
35. D
36. B
37. A
38. B
39. A
40. C

Chapter Four

1. D
2. B
3. D
4. C
5. A
6. D
7. C
8. B
9. D
10. B
11. C
12. D
13. B
14. A
15. A
16. D
17. D
18. B
19. D
20. A
21. D
22. A
23. B
24. C
25. B
26. A

27. D
28. C
29. A
30. C
31. A
32. C
33. D
34. B
35. A
36. D
37. C
38. D
39. B
40. C

Chapter Five

1. B
2. C
3. C
4. A
5. D
6. B
7. C
8. A
9. B
10. C
11. B
12. A
13. D
14. C
15. D
16. D
17. B
18. C
19. D
20. B
21. B
22. C
23. B
24. B
25. D

26. B
27. C
28. C
29. C
30. D
31. D
32. C
33. A
34. C
35. B
36. B
37. A
38. C
39. C
40. B

Chapter Six

1. B
2. C
3. A
4. C
5. A
6. B
7. A
8. A
9. D
10. C
11. A
12. C
13. D
14. A
15. D
16. D
17. B
18. B
19. A
20. C
21. D
22. D
23. C
24. C

25. B
26. D
27. A
28. A
29. B
30. B
31. A
32. C
33. D
34. C
35. B
36. B
37. D
38. C
39. A
40. A

Chapter Seven

Question	Option
1	B
2	B
3	A
4	D
5	B
6	C
7	D
8	C
9	A
10	A
11	B

12	D
13	C
14	A
15	C
16	C
17	B
18	A
19	A
20	C

Question	Option
21	A
22	A
23	B
24	C
25	D
26	A
27	D
28	A
29	C
30	B
31	A
32	D
33	C
34	A
35	B
36	B
37	D
38	C
39	D
40	D

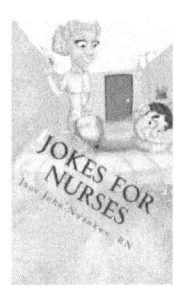 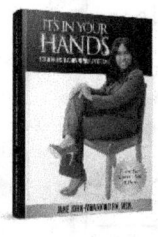 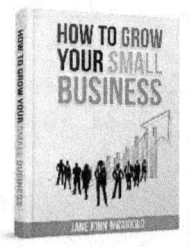 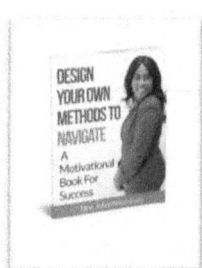 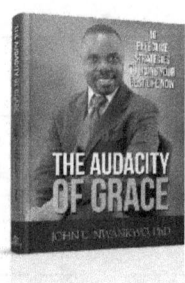

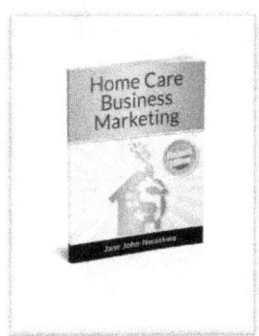 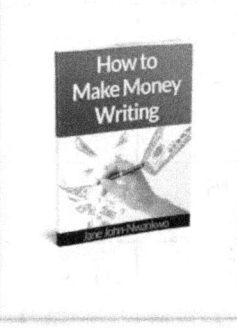 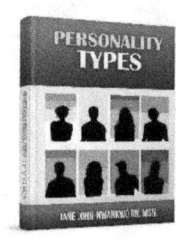 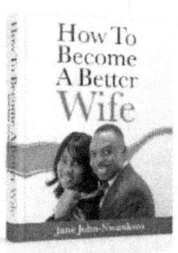

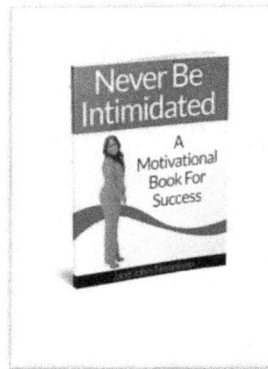 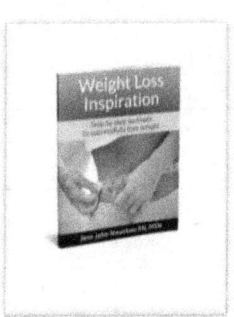 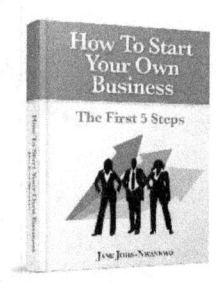 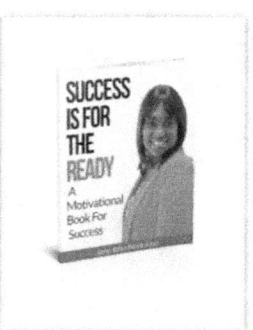

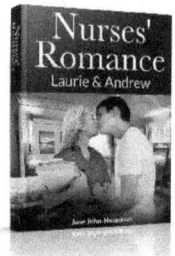 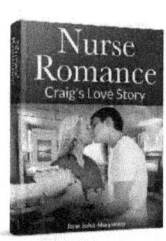 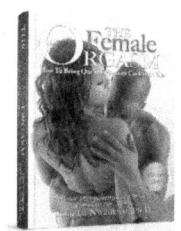 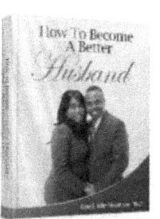

www.janejohn-nwankwo.com   Search books on Amazon.com

ABOUT THE AUTHOR

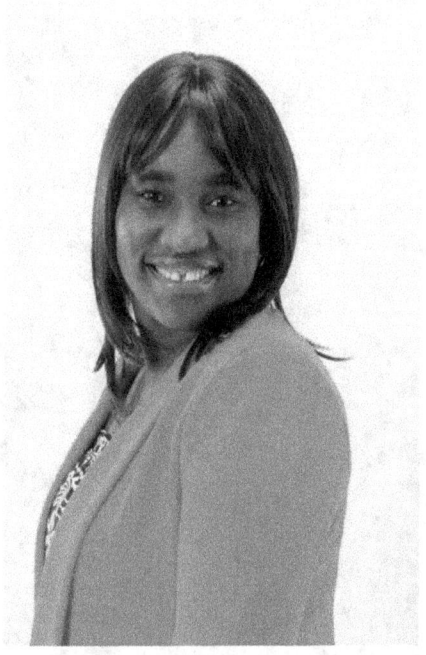

Jane John-Nwankwo CPT, RN, MSN, PHN is a motivational speaker and published author of more than 50 books which include textbooks for healthcare training, fiction for entertainment, and motivational books.

Simply search

"Books by Jane John-Nwankwo"

On Amazon.com

Visit her website:

www.janejohn-nwankwo.com

Book Jane John-Nwankwo as your motivational speaker now at
www.JaneJohn-Nwankwo.com

With more than 10 years as a professional speaker, Jane John-Nwankwo can hold any audience sitting straight on their chairs for any length of time! She is a seminar leader and a published author of more than 50 books including textbooks for healthcare training, fiction for entertainment, books for new entrepreneurs and motivational and inspirational books like the "It's in your hands" series.

She earned her Masters of Science in Nursing from University of Phoenix. She is currently an educational consultant, as well as an entrepreneurial consultant. Her speaking interests include: Motivational speeches for new business owners, Motivational speeches for any category of people, Employee seminars, Students' Empowerment, Healthcare topics, Topics related to women and any Christian topic. Book a speaking appointment today Wow! your audience. Electrify your seminar!!

www.janejohn-nwankwo.com

Having

compassion for the

elderly is a good way

to prepare for one's

own aging

-Jane John-Nwankwo